Black Pepper Essential Oil

Benefits, Properties, Applications, Studies & Recipes

by Ann Sullivan

Published in USA by:

Ann Sullivan
217 N. Seacrest Blvd #9
Boynton Beach
FL 33425

© Copyright 2015

ISBN-13: 978-1545129333
ISBN-10: 1545129339

TABLE OF CONTENTS

Introduction

What are essential oils, and how might they be used for therapeutic purposes?

Essential oils are ultra-potent oils, extracted from plants and flowers that have been utilized in medicine for centuries. Presently, they're most commonly used to supplement pharmaceutical medication, but they can also be an effective alternative to pharmaceuticals in the event that you don't have access to them. Before you dismiss essential oils as a means to support the body's natural defenses against injuries and illness, take a look at the historical evidence of the oils' medicinal competence in practice. Your average age-old medical text will demonstrate that essential oils, herbs, and plenty of other natural ingredients have, for thousands of years, successfully enhanced immune function to meet and defeat any number of ailments and injuries. Though traditional medicine is considered "alternative" now, it was once the gold standard. And, frankly, perhaps it still should be, as these natural age-tested remedies can fortify the body's battlements against everything from simple maladies, like headaches, cuts and bruises, to serious diseases, like cancer.

Essential oils are deemed "essential," because the oils are composed of the "essence" of the plant. The difference between essential oils and other oils – like olive oil or vegetable oil, for instance – is that essential oils have high volatility and reduced fixation, which results in faster evaporation, enabling their popular use in aromatherapy. Even at high temperatures, olive and vegetable oils don't evaporate.

Essential oils are especially necessary when it comes to a major natural or man-made disaster or some potential viral outbreak. In these types of dire situations, you may not have quick access (or any access at all) to your standard pharmaceutical supply; so essential oils, along with other alternative medicines, will be your go-to health aids in the case of social collapse, viral outbreak or devastating natural disaster. When medical access is null and void, alternatives to our modern-day standard are the only chance we have to keep pathogens at bay.

You probably don't realize that you already use essential oils every day. They're in perfumes, shampoos, soaps, ointments...they're even used in furniture polish. Why are they found in so many aromatic products? Well, basically, because essential oils are super concentrated aromatic liquids, so their scent is remarkably strong. Let's put this into perspective: to steam tea, you use a few leaves of peppermint or juniper; to produce a single ounce of essential oil, five whole pounds of peppermint or juniper leaves are required. Some sources claim that to produce twelve pounds of essential oil would necessitate an acre of peppermint, juniper, or any other oil you're looking to produce en masse. Unlike vegetable oil, you don't often find concentrated therapeutic-grade essential oils sold by the tubload; instead the oils are often sold in easily carried small, dark bottles, perfect for your GOOD bag (Get Out Of Dodge). Which is exactly what this book is aiming to help you do – get out of dodge with your most vital of essential oils intact, in particular a good supply of black pepper essential oil.

Why black pepper, you ask? Well, in order to get you quickly up to speed on this most essential of oils, below we've provided a condensed synopsis of black pepper, after which we'll outline in greater detail the oil's history, properties, and common therapeutic uses, so that you – the consumer – might have a better understanding of the oil's benefits and applications. We've even provided supportive remedies for pure cassia, as well as blended recipes that incorporate the valuable oil. Chapter 3 will further detail past scientific research on black pepper essential oil.

Now, let's get down to it – **Essential Oil 101: the Basics of Black pepper.**

Summary: Black Pepper, or Piper nigrum, has been used for hundreds of years in supporting the body's defenses against cholera and malaria. These contagious diseases were fatal to many before water was properly treated. Nowadays, black pepper's most popular uses include supporting the body's defenses against digestive issues, dysentery, nausea, heartburn and even tooth infections. More than 2,000 species of pepper exist and most are not of medicinal quality. Be aware of this when purchasing.

Description: Black Pepper oil is commonly extracted through steam distillation. The peppercorn is most often used. The oil is clear in color, thin in consistency, and has a medium crisp pepper scent.

Uses: Beyond those applications previously mentioned, additional uses for black pepper essential oil include strengthening the body's defenses against flu, dysentery, tooth infections, fungal infections, fatigue, digestive issues, flatulence, diarrhea, constipation, nausea, heartburn, indigestion, colic, sprains, viruses, muscle pain, nerve pain, vomiting, chilblains, poor circulation, and arthritis. It also supports the metabolism and the endocrine system. When it comes to mood and emotion, black pepper can give the user a boost of energy.

Properties: Antioxidant, antiviral, antibacterial, anti-inflammatory, anticatarrhal, antispasmodic, antiseptic, analgesic, laxative, expectorant, digestive, diuretic and carminative properties.

Application: Dilute 1:1 with a carrier oil. You can apply topically, diffuse or use as a dietary supplement.

Safety Precautions: Black pepper has been approved by the FDA for internal consumption and so can be used as a dietary supplement. If you have sensitive skin, dilute heavily and test before extensive use.

Fun facts: Black pepper is so named, because "pippali" in Sanskrit means "long pepper."

The uses of black pepper are so versatile and were once held in such high esteem that the oil can even be found in the tombs of Egyptian kings. Traces of black pepper were discovered in the nostrils and on the abdomen of the mummified body of Ramses II.

Chapter 1:
Benefits of Black pepper Essential Oil

Black pepper essential oil offers a number of therapeutic benefits; but you may be wondering what these benefits are. In this chapter, we'll take a closer look at the history of black pepper and its many uses.

Cultivation of Black Pepper

Black pepper, or Piper nigrum, is a member of the Piperaceae family. The fruit of this flowering vine is cultivated, dried, and often used to season or spice culinary dishes. The perennial pepper plant can grow up to 13 feet tall on support systems, like trellises or poles. The vine spreads and the stems root to the ground, sprouting leaves and flowers, which eventually form the fruit – called a "drupe" or, when dried, a "peppercorn" – that is used to make black pepper.

Native to south India, black pepper has been utilized there for thousands of years in cooking and in traditional medicine and is still prominently cultivated in warm, humid regions in south India. The crop thrives in tropical environments, growing well in soil that is moist, unflooded, and with a good amount of organic matter. In fact, 34% of the global production of pepper comes out of Vietnam, which is presently the crop's largest global cultivator and exporter.

To cultivate the fruit from the pepper plants, both ends of each 40-50 centimeter length of plant are tied to neighboring trees or climbing frames, ranged at around two meter intervals. If trees are used, rough barked trees are preferred to smooth barked trees for climbing, along with plenty of shade cover and air flow. The pepper plant's shoots are cut bi-annually, and manure and leaf mulch are piled on the roots. For the first three years, pepper plants must be watered frequently (every other day) during the dry season, after which, in year four or five, the plant starts bearing fruit and continues to do so for seven years, with one stem bearing up to 30 drupes. The fruit is harvested once those at the base start to redden – this means that the fruit is maturing. The drupes are drained of their pungency and fall from the plant if left to ripen entirely.

To make pepper, the unripe green drupes from the pepper plant are cultivated and quickly boiled in hot water, which cleans and readies them for the drying process. The pepper's cell walls are burst by the heat, and this helps to speed up the sun's drying time, which usually lasts for three or more days. They can also be dried by machine – still a several-day process. Drying the drupes shrinks the pepper's seed and makes them dark and wrinkled. In this dried state, it's referred to as "peppercorn."

After drying, oil or pepper spirit may be extracted from the berries through crushing. Medicine and cosmetics utilize the spirits, while the oil has long been used in ayurvedic massage and also in herbal and beauty products.

These peppercorns contain a single seed and, when they are ground, they're what we use as pepper. What most people don't know is that there are three colors of pepper which refer to three states of the peppercorn. White pepper refers to the seeds of the ripe fruit, green pepper refers to the fruit in its dry, unripe state, and black pepper is, as mentioned, referring to the fruit's cooked, dried and unripe state. The last is used in the making of black pepper essential oil.

As the most traded spice in the world, black pepper also has a long history of use in Europe, with European cuisine incorporating pepper in a variety of dishes. Often combined with salt, this power couple has built a long-standing relationship, standing side-by-side on tabletops the world over.

A History of Black Pepper

The roots of the word "pepper" sprout from the Dravidian word "pippali," meaning "long pepper." This "pippali" was adopted by Latin and Greek language and reinstated as "piper," which referred to black pepper and long pepper in the Roman empire, confusing two different spices as one and the same. Long pepper is cultivated from an entirely different plant than black pepper; but both were referred to as "piper" until Old English designated to black pepper, alone, as "pipor." This is from where our present-day word is derived. However, in the 16th century the word "pepper" was used not only used in reference to the seasoning, but in various metaphorical ways – as in referring to a person's energy or spirit, shortened to "pep" in the 20th century – as well as in literal references to the chili pepper, which again was a completely different plant.

Native to South Asia and India, pepper has been a culinary seasoning since 2 BCE. Known as "black gold," pepper was highly prized and was largely sourced from India and traded so regularly and unwaveringly throughout history that our modern day legal system in the west designates a form of payment for goods or services as "peppercorn rent." Trade, during the early days, was mainly with China. When the British began the East India Trading Company, almost all black pepper traded in North Africa, the Middle East, and Europe, came from India; but prior to, the islands of Malaysia and Indonesia were cultivating and trading as well.

The spices of Southeast Asia – black pepper, in particular – were considered such precious commodities when they first became known in Europe and other areas of the world that attempts to find a sea trading route to China were piloted by the Portuguese. Thus the age of exploration, the discovery of the Americas and the subsequent colonization of many foreign lands – all of this history was influenced by the draw of black pepper, along with a few other valued spices.

In ancient Egypt, black peppercorn was used in the mummification process, shoved into the nostrils of dead pharaohs. No one knows how pepper had found its way to Egypt from Asia, but we know it did, as Ramesses II, in 1213 BCE, enjoyed two big peppercorns up his sniffer for thousands of years.

The Greeks saw black pepper as a hot commodity at the time of its introduction in Greece, around the 4th century BCE. Trade in black pepper arrived by land or via the Arabian Sea. It's unlikely that black pepper was affordable or popular amongst the common folk, as it was less accessible than long pepper.

The Roman Empire saw greater trade in 30 BCE, as the Arabian Sea was now open to the Malabar Coast in India. According to records, somewhere around 120 ships were sent from Rome annually to India, China, and Southeast Asia. The roundtrip took a year, timed perfectly with the monsoon winds to carry the fleet across the Arabian while, on the return trip, the fleet pushed up the

Red Sea and was delivered overland to Alexandria and then across to the Roman Empire. This trade route was dominant for over a millennium. And now that the route for black pepper was shorter than the route for long pepper, the rates flip-flopped. Still, it was an expensive and treasured seasoning, one that continued to be valued even after the great empire fell.

Pepper served as a currency in some cases...and ransom in others. When Alaric the Visigoth overtook Rome in the 5th century, he demanded, in part, 3,000 pounds of pepper. When Rome fell, the trade routes were navigated by the Persians. The Arabs followed. And, though the Early Middle Ages saw the spice trade controlled largely by Islam, Italy came back into play, with Genoa and Venice monopolizing the spice trade, once cargo arrived in the Mediterranean.

In the Middle Ages, pepper was still held in high acclaim and still expensive. With the exorbitant prices and Italy's monopoly over the spice trade, Portugal sought a new route to India, around the southern tip of Africa. Once the Portuguese had established a place on the Arabian sea, they were awarded rights by the 1495 Treaty of Tordesillas to half of the area where the spice trade originated, but their stronghold over the trade was only temporary. The Venetian and Arab trade fleets snuck easily through the Portuguese roadblocks and so then were able to smuggle along the African route and continue their trade along the previously established route. To further the Portuguese decline, the English and the Dutch seized control of pepper ports in the 17th century.

With a boost in the pepper supply came a drop in prices. Now, pepper became more common amongst the commoners, and its uses broadened not only when it came to culinary tastes but also when it come to medicine. Used as a curative medication, black pepper was applied to diarrhea, constipation, earache, hernia, heart disease, indigestion, gangrene, sore throat, insomnia, liver problems, joint pain, sunburn, toothache, tooth decay, and lung disease. Powdered black pepper is used in traditional Indian medicine to relieve cough, congestion and sore throat.

Pepper is still the most traded spice in the world and often accounts for around a quarter of all spice imports annually. Vietnam is now its largest exporter.

Chemical Components

The spice from pepper comes from the fruit and the seed's piperine, which composes anywhere from 4.6% to 9.7% of black pepper's mass. Being that the flavor of pepper can be lost through evaporation and light exposure, containing black pepper in airtight and darkened containers can preserve the spice.

In order to generate the essential oil from the pepper plant's fruit, the resin must be steam distilled. This results in the oil's key chemical components, which are primarily linalool, limonene, pinene, sabinene, and caryophyllene.

Main Properties of Black Pepper Essential Oil

Along with the properties previously mentioned in the introduction, black pepper oil possesses antioxidant, antiviral, antibacterial anti-inflammatory, anticatarrhal, antispasmodic, antiseptic, analgesic, laxative, expectorant, digestive, diuretic and carminative properties. With such a versatile range, black pepper is well equipped to fight off any pathogen in the body's path.

Black pepper, as mentioned, is composed of linalool, limonene, pinene, sabinene, and caryophyllene. These components are what instill the enormously beneficial properties within black pepper essential oil. We'll outline these properties below.

Antioxidant

Anything high in antioxidants – whether fruit, beans, or essential oils – is a powerful advocate for your body. Antioxidants both protect against free radicals and repair their damage. What are free radicals? Free radicals are destructive chemicals that invade your body, produced by substances both inside and out. Some free radicals (or oxidants) form through normal bodily reactions, like inflammation, metabolism and aerobic respiration. Other free radicals form outside the body, but enter it due to exposure. These include harmful pollutants, toxins, smoking, alcohol, X-rays, and UV rays, to name a few.

Although our bodies produce their own antioxidants, these often become damaged as we grow older; thus, introducing antioxidants into our bodies allows these nutrients and enzymes to assist in chemical reactions which destroy the oxidants or free radicals. Black pepper essential oil is a moderate antioxidant, aiming to detox the body of free radicals that lead to disease. See a study that analyzes black pepper's antioxidant properties here.

Antiviral

The antiviral protection that black pepper essential oil grants will essentially empower the immune system, building up a tougher wall of security that most colds, measles or mumps are unlikely to scale. By boosting white blood cell count and function, this immune stimulant will ensure that your body is better prepared to protect against deadly viral infections. See a study that examines black pepper's antiviral properties here.

Antibacterial

Black pepper's antibacterial properties make it a powerful protectant against diseases produced by bacteria, such as oral, digestive and urinary tract bacterial infection. What's great is that, unlike some prescription drugs, black pepper has no ill effects on bodily health or on the healthy natural flora that exists within the stomach and intestines.

Anti-inflammatory

External or internal inflammation can be reduced through the use of black pepper essential oil. For instance, if you or your patient has swollen fingers from arthritis or a swollen knee from a sport's injury, oral application of black pepper essential oil may decrease irritation or redness, while also soothing the pain that accompanies inflammation.

Anti-catarrhal

Catarrhal inflammation occurs when the mucous membranes in the body's airways or cavity are inflamed. This can cause a lot of mucous and white blood cells as the result of an infection. The symptom comes with coughs, the common cold, infections of the ear, adenoids, tonsils and sinus. The phlegm issue can potentially become chronic, so addressing it early on with an anti-catarrhal, like black pepper, is a proactive measure to take towards recovery.

Antispasmodic

The antispasmodic properties of black pepper oil make it beneficial to such surgical processes as colonoscopy, gastroscopy, and intraluminally-applied double-contrast barium enema.

Antiseptic

The antiseptic and disinfectant properties of black

pepper essential oil can be reaped topically, applied directly to wounds, or even through burning; the smoke from the oil may help destroy airborne germs. Internal use will help keep the wounds from becoming infections, while external use will inhibit tetanus.

Analgesic

As an analgesic, black pepper supports pain relief, acting on the central nervous system to fortify the body's natural defenses against inflammation and supporting relief from pain receptor sensation. See a study that supports black pepper's analgesic qualities here.

Laxative

As a laxative, black pepper supplements the body's natural defenses against constipation, by loosening stools and supporting bowel movements.

Expectorant

Throat or respiratory infections can be relieved through the use of black pepper essential oil. Acting as an expectorant, black pepper helps break up and destroy the phlegm and mucus buildup that accompanies sinuses or respiratory infections. Inflamed throat and lungs – and, thus, coughing – can also be relieved through the use of this oil.

Digestive

By boosting the production of absorptive enzymes, the digestibility of nutrients, and the secretion of digestive juices, black pepper essential oil aids the digestive tract significantly, which can make a great impact on the body's overall health by increasing those nutrients absorbed from food.

Carminative

By supporting the reduction of excess gas buildup and/or removal of gas from the intestines, black pepper essential oil provides relief from abdominal pain, excess sweating, and uncomfortable indigestion.

Diuretic

If you're looking to lose water weight and reduce blood pressure, black pepper essential oil is your weight loss enhancing agent. The oil stimulates urination, promoting not only the loss of water weight, but the loss of fats, uric acid, sodium, and other body toxins.

Common Medicinal Uses

Used for hundreds of years in enhancing the body's defenses against cholera and malaria, black pepper essential oil remains a significant immune booster, protecting against a number of modern diseases and ailments. Whether the body is plagued with digestive issues, dysentery, nausea, heartburn or any number of other health problems, black pepper has a lot to offer in the way of supporting a body's overall health.

Digestive Aid

A healthy digestive tract means a healthy body, so maintaining good digestion can make a load of difference in how you feel, as a whole. Your digestive tract is between 25 and 30 feet long. If the length of it is not working properly, then there's a chance that food might get caught up and begin to rot within your body. Black pepper essential oil effectively supports the digestive tracts natural function by helping induce bile flow throughout the digestive organs, which will benefit your overall health.

Respiratory Issues

Black pepper helps calm coughing by ridding the lungs and respiratory tracts of phlegm. Bronchitis, congestion, asthma, and other respiratory issues can be supported with black pepper essential oil, as the oil's anti-inflammatory properties help soothe the respiratory tract. See a study on black pepper's potential uses in respiratory issues here.

Joint Pain Relief

Topical application of black pepper essential oil, with its analgesic and anti-inflammatory properties, can be used to support joint pain relief. Enhancing the body's natural inhibition of inflammation, swelling, and pain, through topical application, black pepper can accelerate the healing process when it comes to wounds or injuries.

Skin Issues

With its antibacterial and antifungal properties, black pepper essential oil promotes healthy, glowing skin by enhancing the body's natural healing process, when it comes to skin issues. The oil supports the body in combating bacterial growth.

Oral Hygiene

The antiseptic properties in black pepper essential oil make it an strengthening aid for oral hygiene. Antiseptics destroy bad breath bacteria and also eliminate plaque. On top of that, the oil can help reduce gum bleeding and maintain the mouth's overall health and cleanliness.

Weight loss

Those who need an extra boost to lose unwanted body fat can pop some black pepper essential oil, which has been shown to enhance weight loss and help burn fat. As a diuretic, black pepper supports the body's natural function in reducing water weight and blood pressure. The oil stimulates urination, promoting the loss of fats, uric acid, sodium, and other body toxins.

Safety Precautions & Common Applications

Safety

Some adverse effects may evolve when using pure essential oils. Some essential oils should not be used when pregnant, for example, as they may cause miscarriage. Allergic reactions, too, may occur, especially when applied topically. Always administer an allergy test before committing fully to topical application. When used with other medications, essential oils may react negatively. If you are on any current prescription medications or have a chronic illness, such as high blood pressure, epilepsy or liver disease, then researching the effects of essential oils against your own personal medical history will eliminate any potentially problematic issues.

Black pepper has been approved by the FDA for internal consumption and so can be used as a dietary supplement. If you have sensitive skin, dilute heavily and test before extensive use. Dilute 1:1 with a carrier oil. You can apply topically, diffuse or use as a dietary supplement.

Blends

Oftentimes, essential oils are manufactured as blends of several pure oils. For instance, doTerra's On Guard Essential Oil Blend is a mix of cinnamon, clove, rosemary, and eucalyptus. This blend can be used to boost the immune system to help support colds, viruses and flus. The downside to blends is that the more oils added to the mix, the higher the probability your patient may react negatively to the blend if he/she is prone to allergies. There is also the possibility of phototoxicity when working with blends.

Regardless of these possible effects, essential oils are a viable option for supporting a number of conditions. Those looking to support or maintain their own personal health, or that of their family's, should become educated on the uses of essential oils, their natural remedies and the methods of application. Only then can you begin building your kit of essential oils for survival.

Chapter 2:
Recipes for Black Pepper Essential Oil

In this chapter, we'll offer various recipes for black pepper essential oil, both for pure black pepper applications and blends. For pure applications, we've provided the appropriate application and dosage to support specific ailments, from addiction to viral infections. When it comes to blends, herbalists and aromatherapists often combine black pepper essential oil with lemon, lime, orange, bergamot, myrrh, sandalwood, pine, lavender and benzoin. We'll offer some fantastic blending options in the second half of this chapter.

Pure Applications

Addiction

To help combat addiction, dilute black pepper essential oil in a 1:1 ratio with a carrier oil and apply topically, massaging over the solar plexus and the heart. You can also administer aromatically, diffusing throughout the home or inhaling directly from the bottle. See a study that supports black pepper's application in addiction here.

Arthritis

Support the body's natural defenses against the pain and inflammation of arthritis by diluting black pepper essential oil in a 1:1 ratio with a carrier oil and apply topically, massaging the oil into the joints.

Back or Neck Pain

To help ease lower back pain or neck pain, place four drops of black pepper essential oil onto a hot compress. Let the compress rest on the affected until it reaches your body temperature. Reapply as needed.

Blood Circulation

Boost blood circulation by diffusing black pepper essential oil throughout the home. You can also apply topically by diluting black pepper essential oil in a 1:1 ratio with a carrier oil and massaging the oil into the affected area.

Cellular Oxygenation

To help increase oxygen to the brain, administer aromatically. Pour a drop into your hands, rub your palms together, cup them over your nose, and breathe, or you can simply diffuse throughout the home.

Chills

If you're feeling the chills, dilute black pepper essential oil in a 1:1 ratio with a carrier oil and apply topically, massaging the oil into the soles of the feet.

Colds

Combat the common cold by diffusing black pepper essential oil throughout the home. You can also apply topically by diluting black pepper essential oil in a 1:1 ratio with a carrier oil and massaging into the chest and the soles of the feet.

Constipation

To help relieve constipation, dilute black pepper essential oil in a 1:1 ratio with a carrier oil and massage in a clockwise motion over the abdomen.

Cough

Treat a cough by diffusing black pepper essential oil

throughout the home or inhaling directly from the bottle. You can also dilute black pepper essential oil in a 1:1 ratio with a carrier oil and apply topically, massaging into the throat, chest and the soles of the feet. A fourth option is to gargle a couple drops of the oil in 4-5 ounces of water.

Diarrhea

If you're experiencing diarrhea, black pepper essential oil is a superb support. Apply topically by diluting the oil in a 1:1 ratio with a carrier oil and massaging it into the abdomen in a counterclockwise motion, or place a drop of the oil in your drinking water throughout the day.

Digestion

To aid digestion, place a drop in your drinking water or incorporate into your cooking. You can also apply topically by diluting black pepper essential oil in a 1:1 ratio with a carrier oil and massaging it into the abdomen.

Emotional Balance

Black pepper essential oil can help provide emotional balance by diluting 1 drop of peppermint essential oil in 1 tablespoon of a carrier oil and apply topically, massaging into the chest. You can also administer the oil aromatically by diffusing or inhaling directly from the bottle.

Energy

To give yourself a spurt of energy, dilute black pepper essential oil in a 1:1 ratio with a carrier oil and apply topically, massaging into the soles of the feet. You can also diffuse throughout the room or inhale directly from the bottle.

Flatulence

Relieve gas by diluting black pepper essential oil in a 1:1 ratio with a carrier oil and massaging into the abdomen in a clockwise motion. You can also place a drop in a glass of water and take orally.

Flu

Support your body's natural defenses against the flu by diluting black pepper essential oil in a 1:1 ratio with a carrier oil and massaging it into sore muscles and joints, into the reflex points of the feet, or over the abdominal area, if you're experiencing diarrhea. You can also diffuse throughout the home to support general health during cold/flu season.

Immune System

Give your immune system a leg up by regularly diffusing black pepper throughout your home, especially during cold and flu season. The scent also uplifts and boosts energy. Alternatively, you can add a couple drops to your bathwater or dilute with a carrier oil and apply topically, massaging it into the soles of the feet. If you'd prefer the steam method, steam two drops of black pepper essential oil in a pan of water, remove the steaming pan from the stove, pour into a bowl, place a towel over your head and inhale. If you don't feel it's done its job the first time, you can reheat that same water and use it once more without adding more oil.

Loss of Appetite

If grief, stress, illness, or depression causes you to experience appetite loss, diffuse black pepper essential oil throughout the home. You can also dilute the oil in a 1:1 ratio with a carrier oil and apply topically, massaging into the stomach before each meal.

Neuralgia

Neuralgia and the pain caused by neuralgia can be relieved by diluting black pepper essential oil in a 1:1 ratio with a carrier oil and massaging it over the affected area once daily.

Stroke

Enhance the body's defenses against stroke by diffusing black pepper essential oil throughout the home or inhaling directly.

Toothache

To help alleviate toothache, dilute 1 drop of black pepper essential oil with 1 teaspoon coconut oil and apply topically to the affected area.

Vertigo

Combat vertigo and maintain balance by diffusing black pepper essential oil throughout the home. You can also pour a drop into your hands, rub your palms together, cup them over your nose, and breathe deeply for thirty seconds.

Viral Infections

Strengthen your body's defenses against viral infections by diluting black pepper essential oil with a carrier oil and massaging into the reflex points of the feet. You can also place a few drops in your bathwater or diffuse throughout the home

Vomiting

To help stave off vomiting, place a drop of black pepper essential oil in your drinking water. You can apply topically, diluting the oil in a 1:1 ratio with a carrier oil and apply topically, massaging it into the abdomen and into the reflex points of the feet. You can also inhale directly or diffuse throughout the home.

Warming

Enhance body warmth by diluting black pepper essential oil in a 1:1 ratio with a carrier oil and massaging it into the reflex points of the feet.

Blends

Aphrodisiac

Ingredients

- 1 drop Ylang Ylang Essential Oil
- 1 drop Black Pepper Essential Oil
- 1 drop Rose Otto Essential Oil
- 1 Tbsp Sweet Almond Oil

Directions

In a small bowl or container, mix all ingredients until well combined. Warm slightly then to help relax and relieve sore muscles, apply in a full-body massage.

Constipation Relief

Ingredients

- 1 drop Lavender Essential Oil

- 1 drop Black Pepper Essential Oil

- 1 drop Sweet Marjoram Essential Oil

- 1 Tbsp Sweet Almond Oil

Directions

In a small bowl or container, mix all ingredients until well combined. Massage in a clockwise motion into the lower abdomen. Also massage into the shoulders, neck and back.

Constipation Relief II

Ingredients

- 5 drops Black Pepper Essential Oil

- 5 drops Cardamom Essential Oil

- 15 drops Patchouli Essential Oil

- 2 Tbsps Sweet Almond Oil

Directions

In a small bowl or container, mix all ingredients until well combined. Massage in a clockwise motion into the lower abdomen. Also massage into the shoulders, neck and back.

De-stress Bath

Ingredients

- 2 drops Rosemary Essential Oil

- 3 drops Black Pepper Essential Oil

- 5 drops Grapefruit Essential Oil

- 1 Tbsp Grapeseed Oil

Directions

To wind down, de-stress, and combat anxiety, add all ingredients to your bathwater and stir to disperse. Then inhale deeply while you soak for 20 minutes, but avoid getting water in your eyes, as it may sting.

Energy Booster

Ingredients

- 10 drops Orange Essential Oil

- 10 drops Cinnamon Essential Oil

- 10 drops Black Pepper Essential Oil

Directions

Diffuse blend throughout your home to stimulate energy.

Fallen Arches

Ingredients

- 5 drops Black Pepper Essential Oil

- 5 drops Clary Sage Essential Oil

- 10 drops Ginger Essential Oil

- 10 drops Rosemary Essential Oil

- 2 Tsp Carrier Oil

Directions

To relieve the stress of fallen arches, combine all ingredients in a small bowl, blending well. Apply to the instep of the foot, massaging toward the heel.

Focused Concentration

Ingredients

- 3 drops Black Pepper Essential Oil
- 3 drops Ginger Essential Oil
- 3 drops Cardamom Essential Oil
- 3 drops Basil Essential Oil

Directions

To help focus concentration, diffuse throughout the home or office.

Muscle Relief

Ingredients

- 3 drops Black Pepper Essential Oil
- 3 drops Pine Essential Oil
- 4 drops Lavender Essential Oil
- 5 drops Niaouli Essential Oil
- 15 mL Carrier Oil

Directions

In a small bowl or container, mix all ingredients until well combined. Warm slightly then to help relax and relieve sore muscles, apply in a full-body massage.

Muscle Relief II

Ingredients

- 12 drops Black Pepper Essential Oil
- 6 drops Ginger Essential Oil
- 6 drops Marjoram Essential Oil
- 6 drops Juniper Berry Essential Oil
- 8 ounces Sweet Almond Oil

Directions

In a small bowl or container, mix all ingredients until well combined. Warm slightly then to help relax and relieve sore muscles, apply in a full-body massage.

Osteoarthritis

Ingredients

- 4 drops Cedarwood Essential Oil

- 5 drops Cypress Essential Oil

- 8 drops Black Pepper Essential Oil

- 13 drops Ginger Essential Oil

- 2 Tbsps Almond Oil

Directions

To help relieve the pain and swelling caused by osteoarthritis, combine all ingredients in a small bowl, blending well. Apply topically, massaging into the affected area.

Peritonsillar Abscess

Ingredients

- 1 drop Black Pepper Essential Oil
- 1 drop Lemon Essential Oil
- 5 ounces Water

Directions

Combine ingredients and mix well. Gargle mixture 3-4 times throughout the day.

Rubbing Oil for Painful Joints

Ingredients

- 1 cup Carrier Oil

- 2 drops Black Pepper Essential Oil

- 4 drops Cajuput Essential Oil

- 8 drops Eucalyptus Essential Oil

- 10 drops Marjoram Essential Oil

Directions

Combine all ingredients in a glass jar or dropper bottle. Place the lid on and shake vigorously to combine. Apply by massaging gently into sore muscles and joints.

Strained Arm

Ingredients

- 5 drops Black Pepper Essential Oil
- 5 drops Nutmeg Essential Oil
- 20 drops Ginger Essential Oil
- 2 Tbsps Almond Oil

Directions

Relieve arm strain by combining all ingredients in a small bowl, blending well. Massage into the affected area three times a day until you feel relief.

Strained Neck

Ingredients

- 5 drops Black Pepper Essential Oil

- 5 drops Peppermint Essential Oil

- 10 drops Ginger Essential Oil

- 10 drops Rosemary Essential Oil

- 2 Tbsps Almond Oil

Directions

Relieve neck strain by combining all ingredients in a small bowl, blending well. Massage into the affected area three times a day until you feel relief.

Warming Massage

Ingredients

- 2 drops Ginger Essential Oil

- 3 drops Black Pepper Essential Oil

- 5 drops Sandalwood Essential Oil

- 15 drops Ylang Ylang Essential Oil

- 15 mL Carrier Oil

Directions

In a small bowl or container, mix all ingredients until well combined. Warm slightly then to help relax and relieve sore muscles, apply in a full-body massage.

Chapter 3:
Black Pepper Essential Oil Studies

Many studies have been done on essential oils to discover and prove their therapeutic qualities. In the case of the great number of black pepper studies, many of the properties attributed to the essential oil (noted in this book and elsewhere) are quite often validated through the scientific research of accredited universities and published by accredited scientific journals. In this chapter, we'll discuss a small portion of these studies. It's important to note that research on essential oils is constant and evolving. Keep up with any recent research, as it may turn up even further valuable uses of these miracle oils.

Study 1 – Neck Pain

In this study available on PubMed, the analgesic effects of black pepper essential oil on neck pain were examined, with the following results: "To assess the efficacy of aromatic essential oils on neck pain...The essential oil cream developed in this study can be used to improve neck pain."

The study observed sixty participants with a neck disability index (NDI) of greater than 10%. Half of the participants were placed in a control group and the other half in an experimental group. The participants in the experimental group were provided a cream to apply to their necks after showering or bathing. The 2 grams of cream was composed of black pepper, lavender, marjoram, and peppermint. Throughout the duration of the study, pain was assessed through a visual analogue scale (VAS), through the pressure pain threshold (PPT), and the neck-joint range was analyzed via a motion analysis system (MAS).

Though VAS scores improved for both the control and experimental groups, the experimental group's pain tolerance improved significantly, according to PPT, NDI and MAS results. In fact the MAS results showed that the experimental group experienced great improvement in the 10 motion areas, which indicates that the essential oil cream effectively supports the body's natural defenses against pain.

Reference
http://www.ncbi.nlm.nih.gov/pubmed/25192562]

Study 2 – Antiviral Properties

In this study available on PubMed, the antiviral effects of black pepper essential oil were examined, with the following results: "The long-term usage of antibiotics has resulted in the evolution of multidrug-resistant bacteria. Unlike antibiotics, anti-virulence approaches target bacterial virulence without affecting cell viability, which may be less prone to develop drug resistance...In this study, anti-biofilm screening of 83 essential oils showed that black pepper, cananga, and myrrh oils and their common constituent cis-nerolidol at 0.01 % markedly inhibited S. aureus biofilm formation...This study is one of the most extensive on anti-virulence screening using diverse essential oils and provides comprehensive data on the subject. This finding implies other beneficial effects of essential oils and suggests that black pepper, cananga, and myrrh oils have potential use as anti-virulence strategies against persistent S. aureus infections."

This study tested the antibacterial and antiviral properties of black pepper against Staphylococcus aureus. Staphylococcus aureus is a Gram-positive bacterium. Although Staphylococcus aureus is part of the normal human skin flora and respiratory tract and is not typically pathogenic, when it becomes so, S. aureus produces respiratory issues like sinusitis, skin infections, and even food poisoning. Those with compromised immune systems are particularly vulnerable to the bacteria and can potentially develop an infection.

According to the study, three of the essential oils tested – including black pepper essential oil – completely inhibited the activity of S. aureus at below 0.005%. Black pepper was the only oil to down-regulate (aka, reduce cellular response to a molecule, by decreasing the number of receptors on the cell surface) the expressions of the nuclease genes, α-toxin gene (hla), and the regulatory genes. Essentially, the study demonstrated that black pepper and other essential oils may be alternative substitutes when bacteria becomes resistant to antibiotics.

Reference
http://www.ncbi.nlm.nih.gov/pubmed/25027570]

Study 3 – Diabetes/Hypertension

In this study published by Advances in Pharmacological Sciences, the effects of black pepper essential oil on diabetes and hypertension were examined, with the following results: "The antioxidant properties and effect of essential oil of black pepper (Piper guineense) seeds on α -amylase, α -glucosidase (key enzymes linked to type-2 diabetes), and angiotensin-I converting enzyme (ACE) (key enzyme linked to hypertension) were assessed...Conclusively, the phenolic content, antioxidant activity, and inhibition of α -amylase, α -glucosidase, and angiotensin-1 converting enzyme activities by the essential oil extract of black pepper could be part of the mechanism by which the essential oil could manage and/or prevent type-2 diabetes and hypertension."

This study analyzed the effects of black pepper essential oil on enzymes related to type-2 diabetes and hypertension. α -amylase and α -glucosidase are both enzymes, largely prevalent in saliva and pancreatic fluid. They convert glycogen, starch, and other complex carbohydrates, into simple sugars. Angiotensin-1 is a peptide hormone that increases blood pressure by inducing vasoconstriction.

Black pepper essential oil was shown to inhibit α -amylase, α -glucosidase, and ACE enzyme activities, with a stronger inhibition of α –glucosidase activities than α -amylase. These results indicate that the antioxidant activity of the oil, alongside the oil's capacity to inhibit α -amylase, α -glucosidase, and angiotensin-1, could make black pepper essential oil supplementary to treatment and prevention of type-2 diabetes and hypertension.

Reference
http://www.ncbi.nlm.nih.gov/pubmed/24348547
http://www.ncbi.nlm.nih.gov/pmc/articles/PMC3856121/pdf/APS2013-926047.pdf

Study 4 – Nicotine Addiction

In this study available on PubMed, the effects of black pepper essential oil on nicotine addiction were examined, with the following results: "To evaluate the effect of two inhaled essential oils (black pepper or angelica) on the nicotine habits of students, staff, and faculty on a U.S. college campus...Both black pepper and angelica reduced the level of nicotine craving and allowed a longer delay before next use of tobacco. However, black pepper reduced the level of craving more than did angelica, and angelica allowed for a longer delay than did black pepper...Aromatherapy may be useful in nicotine withdrawal. Further studies are warranted."

This study was a comparative analysis of the effects of angelica and black pepper essential oil, measured by pre- and post-test results recorded by a sample of 20 regular nicotine users. The participants used either chewing tobacco, snuff, or cigarettes on a daily basis. The participants inhaled one drop of essential oil from a tissue for two minutes whenever they felt a nicotine craving coming on. The participants then self-assessed their level of craving pre-inhalation and post-inhalation on a scale from 0-10, and also recorded the amount of time the inhalation worked – that is, how long it took the participant to crave and use tobacco again.

The results indicated that aromatherapy can, in fact, be applied to nicotine withdrawal. Angelica and black pepper both reduced nicotine cravings and delayed tobacco use.

Black pepper, in particular, was shown to reduce the level of craving at a higher rate than angelica.

Reference
http://www.ncbi.nlm.nih.gov/pubmed/23536963

Study 5 – Vein Visibility

In this study published by the Indian Journal of Pharmaceutical Sciences, the effects of black pepper essential oil on vein visibility were examined, with the following results: "To evaluate the effect of topically applied black pepper essential oil on easing intravenous catheter insertion (IVC) in patients with no palpable or visible veins compared to a control group (standard nursing practice)...A higher percentage of patients achieved optimal scoring (vein score=2) or improved scoring (vein score of 1 or 2) to black pepper intervention than standard nursing care. The black pepper group also reduced the number of patients whose veins were still not visible or palpable after the intervention to nearly half that of the control group ($p < 0.05$). The number of IVC attempts following black pepper was also half that of the control group...Topical application of black pepper is a viable and effective way to enhance vein visibility and palpability prior to intravenous insertion in patients with limited vein accessibility; it also improves ease of IVC insertion."

This study took a look at 120 hospital patients, whose veins were difficult to access for IVC insertion. The patients were divided into a control group and an experimental group. The control group received standard nursing care, which generally includes hot packs, while the experimental group received a topical application composed of 80% aloe vera gel and 20% black pepper essential oil. The pre- and post-test vein visibility were then recorded, as well as the attempts at IVC insertion.

The topical application of black pepper and aloe vera improved vein visibility and IVC insertion by nearly double that of the control group. These results demonstrate the efficacy of black pepper essential oil in intravenous insertion for those with difficult vein accessibility.

Reference
http://www.ncbi.nlm.nih.gov/pubmed/23153036
http://www.ncbi.nlm.nih.gov/pmc/articles/PMC3309643/

Study 6 – Pneumonia Symptoms

In this study published by the Department of Pharmacognosy at Mansoura University in Egypt, the effects of olfactory stimulation by black pepper essential oil were examined, with the following results: "To determine the effect of olfactory stimulation with volatile black pepper oil (BPO) on risk factors for pneumonia...Inhalation of BPO, which can activate the insular or orbitofrontal cortex, resulting in improvement of the reflexive swallowing movement, might benefit older poststroke patients with dysphagia regardless of their level of consciousness or physical and mental status."

This study was a random, controlled study, lasting the duration of a month, that analyzed 105 poststroke residents at a long-term care facility. Pre- and post-study measurements were recorded, including the number of swallowing movements, the regional cerebral blood flow (rCBF), the latency of the swallowing reflex (LTSR) and the serum substance P (SP).

The study showed that black pepper essential oil improved measurements across the board, which indicates that the reflexive swallowing movement can be improved in severely limited patients, like poststroke patients, through the inhalation of black pepper essential oil.

Reference
http://www.ncbi.nlm.nih.gov/pubmed/16970649]

Chapter 4:
The Ins & Outs of Essential Oils

Where do essential oils come from?

Plants and plant species naturally produce essential oils for various reasons, one being to draw pollinator insects to them, another being to repel invading organisms (bacteria, animals). A number of chemical compounds compose each plant's essential oil, and the combination of these compounds is specific to each oil, which then instills in the oil its own unique properties. Essential oils can be harnessed from all sorts of plant components, including flowers, leaves, bark, fruit, roots, and resin. For instance, cinnamon oil is harnessed from bark, lemon oil from the peel, and lavender oil from lavender flowers. Certain plants can produce a few chemical variants of the same essential oil, which are acquired from different parts of the plant.

Some of these parts produce a large amount of oil, while others produce just a smidgen. The oil's quality and potency depends upon a number of factors, including the subspecies of the plant, its soil conditions, the time of year and even the time of day you harvest it.

How are essential oils extracted?

Essential oils can be extracted from plants through various methods, including pressing, distillation, solvent and maceration. Let's take a brief look at each:

Pressing Method

Commonly used with citrus fruit, the pressing method extracts the oil through a technique which involves pushing the fruit peels through a press. Oily fruits and plants are best suited for this technique. Orange oil, for example, is extracted from orange skins through the pressing method.

Distillation Method

This technique harkens back to the days of old-timey moonshiners, as the same sort of method used to create strong liquor can be used to extract essential oils. Using a still, boiled water and plant materials will create steam which is then cooled by coils and condensed into a combination of water and oil. This combination doesn't mix, so the oil can then be extracted from it.

Solvent Method

Through a multi-step process, certain plant and flower oils can be extracted using alcohol and other solvents, which extort the essential oil from the plant materials.

Maceration Method

When a "carrier" or fixed oil or lard is mixed with the plant material and set out in the sun, over a period of time, the carrier oil is infused with the plant's essence. Heat sources, other than the sun, are often used to speed the process. Throughout the process, more plant material is added to produce a more potent oil.

How do you use essential oils?

Although some studies about the effectiveness of essential oils are conducted by small companies or even individuals, a number of them are conducted by the food and cosmetic industries. In general, the pharmaceutical industry shows next to no interest in herbal medicine, primarily because there are few options to patent such products. Being as such, the product's lack of profitability results in a lack of research funding. Regardless, the historical uses of essential oils tell us what we need to know: these oils have been effectively administered for centuries. The therapeutic qualifications of essential oils can be plotted in the survival of the human race across cultures and generations.

Another reason that studies on essential oils have not resulted in much conclusive evidence as to their overall effectiveness is because definitive results are sometimes difficult to prove, as the quality of each batch of oil can vary for a number of reasons. One is that essential oils are impossible to standardize. As mentioned above, even the slightest variance in soil conditions and the time of harvesting – as well as innumerable other factors – will produce a different product quality and potency. In addition, essential oils are often obtained from various species of the same plant; Eucalyptus radiata and Eucalyptus globulus can both be used in the making of therapeutic-grade eucalyptus oil and, as a result, they may have slightly different properties and degrees of strength or effectiveness.

Just as there are a number of methods by which to extract essential oils, there are a number of methods to administer them therapeutically. The variety of chemical compounds in each essential oil means that their benefits and applications also vary across the board. Below are a few of these methods.

Topical Administration

Direct application of many essential oils works like a sponge, as skin sops up chemicals and other things (like sunlight, for instance). Topical application is best when you want to clear up an ailment on the skin's surface or in the underlying muscle tissue. When applying topically, you may either massage the oil into the skin or simply dab on the skin for therapeutic results. You might combine the essential oil with a carrier oil for topical use in order to dilute its potency. This is safer, as the oil is so concentrated. You may support your body's defenses against rash or muscle pain in this manner, but you should always test your patient for allergies before applying. Adverse effects are produced by natural chemicals as much as synthetic ones; poison ivy, for example.

To test for allergens, place a drop or two on your patient's inner forearm. If a rash develops within 12 to 24 hours, then the patient is allergic. In addition, phototoxicity – sun exposure resulting in an exacerbated burn – may be an issue when citrus oils are applied topically. So one must proceed with caution when applying essential oils using this method.

Inhalation Therapy

Commonly known as "aromatherapy", this essential oil application is effective for inner ailments, like sore throat or cold. In a steaming bowl of distilled or sterilized water, add a few drops of essential oil and, with a towel over your head, bend over the bowl and inhale. The towel captures the vapors, making the technique even more effective. Essential oils can also be placed in a diffuser or potpourri throughout a room to produce somewhat diluted therapeutic effects.

Ingestion

When using this method, proceed with caution. Direct ingestion of essential oils must be monitored and applied in small doses that are diluted in a tablespoon or more of any carrier oil – olive oil, for example. If you are unsure of dosage amounts, make a tea with the relevant herb instead. Although the effects of this diluted use may be weaker, this application is a better alternative than an overdose of essential oils.

What are the general benefits of using essential oils?

Replacement for Prescription Drugs

One practical benefit for using essential oils is, of course, their substitutive nature; they can replace Rx drugs, which is the ultimate reason to educate yourself on their administration and to begin stockpiling your essential oil supply. One of the potential threats of economic or social collapse is the lack of resources, and primarily the inability to procure prescription drugs. Being as such, finding suitable supplements should be a priority when preparing for the worst.

Their portability is also a major bonus when it comes to survival prepping. The fact that these ultra-concentrated oils take up little-to-no space makes toting them to your shelter all the simpler should the need arise. And, because essential oils are highly concentrated, the application used in most methods of administration requires only a drop or two of oil, which means that tiny bottle will be long-lasting.

Cost Effective Supplement

Though money may be the last thing on your mind when it comes to prepping for a survival situation (money may even be obsolete in the event of social collapse), it is worth noting that the expense of essential oils pales in comparison to prescription drugs. Essential oils are a cost effective supplement to prescription medicine.

No Expiration Date

Another benefit of essential oils is that they do not expire, neither do they have "proper storage" requirements. A number of medicines and medicinal products must be replaced every couple years, so this sets essential oils ahead of the pack when it comes to shelf life.

Versatility

Essential oils also offer great versatility. Apart from providing therapeutic benefits, essential oils can be repurposed for household and hygienic applications. For instance, if you're looking for something that might serve your dental hygiene needs in a time of crisis, the protective oil blend is your go-to essential oil. If you want to maintain your skin's tone and condition, frankincense and lavender will do the trick; the latter also serves as sunscreen, so you can inhibit sun damage as well.

When it comes to the house or shelter, you can use essential oils to deodorize, which will come in handy in a disaster scenario where things might start to smell fishy due to lack of proper utilities and care. For example, after the 2011 tsunami and the subsequent nuclear reactor meltdown in Japan, a nurse named Risa Nakahira used essential oils to deodorize and sanitize putrid public bathrooms in overpopulated evacuation facilities. As relief workers searched for survivors, often wading through debris and decay, Nakahira also deodorized their boots and masks using essential oils. The possibilities of these natural oils are endless.

They are also versatile when it comes to the range of patients they're capable of supporting. The wellness of everyone from your great grandfather to your infant baby can be fortified with the aid of essential oils in the appropriate dosage. They even come in handy when supporting the wellness of livestock or pets. From teething infants to dementia in the elderly, from teenagers with acne to dogs with urinary tract infections, essential oils can serve any patient with nearly any ailment.

Conclusion

Now that you know all about what black pepper essential oil can do for you – where it originates, how it's extracted, its benefits and properties, and the different methods of administration – you can use it confidently to support the body's defenses against health issues and start to assemble a kit of essential oils for survival. Essential oils can be purchased online or at your local holistic treatment store. If you intend to stock up through online sources, you might try EssentialSurvival.org or other like sites. We always recommend doTerra brand, as the brand guarantees high quality therapeutic grade oils.

The various benefits of essential oils and their properties are countless. To build your own kit, first focus on acquiring the essential oils which may bear more relevance to your health issues or the potential health threats within your environment. In the event of a viral outbreak, for instance, black pepper essential oil will be one of your more crucial oils – along with oregano, lemon, frankincense and cinnamon (eBooks also available for purchase) – due to their antiviral and immuno-supportive properties.

Used as a supplement or as your go-to for arthritis treatment, vertigo balance, or immune-boosting agents, the application of black pepper essential oil in medicine has survived for centuries and will survive centuries more.

When it comes down to it, you don't need to rely on pharmaceuticals; essential oils, herbs, and plenty of other natural ingredients can be used to help treat any number of health issues, whether ailment or injury.

Essential oils are essential to your survival in the case of viral outbreak, social collapse or natural disaster because, when the SHTF, your access to pharmaceuticals will likely either be limited or eliminated altogether. Alternatives to our modern-day standard will equate survival when no other option exists. And when it comes to a life-or-death situation, you can't let your health decline, no matter the state of the world.

DISCLAIMER AND/OR LEGAL NOTICES: Every effort has been made to accurately represent this book and it's potential. Results vary with every individual, and your results may or may not be different from those depicted. No promises, guarantees or warranties, whether stated or implied, have been made that you will produce any specific result from this book. Your efforts are individual and unique, and may vary from those shown. Your success depends on your efforts, background and motivation.

The material in this publication is provided for educational and informational purposes only and is not intended as medical advice. The information contained in this book should not be used to diagnose or treat any illness, metabolic disorder, disease or health problem. Always consult your physician or healthcare provider before beginning any nutrition or exercise program. Use of the programs, advice, and information contained in this book is at the sole choice and risk of the reader.